BAD DAD

By Edward James

I would like to dedicate this book to my amazing wife, family and friends. Without whom I may not be here today to tell my story in the hope to Offer help to others.

CONTENTS

SETTING THE SCENE

I had a very normal, middle class upbringing in the countryside in England. A solid family unit with a nice house, good schools, holidays and an abundance of love. I was brought up to be kind, helpful and honest. My mother did a sterling job especially as she raised me and my siblings from when I was fourteen when my father left us. This naturally had a deep and prolonged effect on me and the family but taught me how to be independent, resourceful and proactive from a young age. It also gave me the foundations of what a good and bad relationship is and how you should treat those close to you. Seeing my father lie pathologically and cheat on my mother would make me know exactly what I did not want from a relationship.

This solid upbringing with firm but fair parenting has provided me with a highly accurate moral compass, natural integrity and, ultimately, made me into a decent human being. I am a son, a father, and a husband of which I put my all into. The story you are about to read will highlight how much all of your self can be tested and how resilient humans can be when they need to be. It highlights that no matter how dark things get, there is always a light at the end of the tunnel.

After completing schooling at eighteen I travelled briefly before starting, and not completing, university where I found myself uncomfortable with the reality of getting into debt without an income. This spurred me to leave and find work in a local hospital. This was immediately rewarding both financially and personally. I enjoyed helping others and having a direct impact on people's lives. After a couple of years I thought about studying nursing but was not in a financial position to do so. I was in a relationship which was good at the time but, with hindsight, was not particularly healthy and was not meant to last. During this time I decided to become a police officer which opened up a whole new world of friendships, experiences, a better income and helped me grow as a person. My relationship ended soon after and we left on good terms.

It was 2004 and I was training in my local gym when I was introduced to a girl. We were both single and I was pursued by a mutual friend to ask her out. I was not particularly interested in her but due to being lonely and not knowing what lay in store, I asked her out for a drink. Due to my inexperience in relationships and inner want to start a "home" with someone we started dating. Initially I was in awe of an older woman of eight years and we entered into a relationship. This was flawed from the outset with a mis match of minds, personalities, opinions and wants from life. Despite this we decided to move in in together and create a home. The relationship was fractious with constant arguments and misunderstandings which, again with hindsight, should have been a great big alarm bell ringing to run for the hills but I clearly had a lesson to be learned.

Throughout our time together I felt undervalued, taken for granted, not listened to, controlled and micromanaged for the entirety. This was only exacerbated after having children. Looking back, this cumulative behaviour surmounted to abusive behaviour which stifled my personality and life in so many ways. Little did I know at the time what this individual was capable of.

The next few years passed and it was obvious to all but us that our fragmented relationship which saw infidelity, break ups, relentless arguments, lack of trust, jealousy and unhappiness was flawed. Despite this, we pressed on in the hope that things would improve and subsequently married. There were, of course, good times but these are now significantly marred. This should have been a sign for both of us to call is a day.

After deciding to leave the police after a few years I returned to my interest working in hospitals. This lead to me successfully getting a place at university to study adult nursing. This coincided with us having our first child leaving my wife unable to work. Having a keen interest in fitness, I qualified as a personal trainer and started my own business whilst studying full time, working hospital placements, being a new dad and trying to keep our heads above water financially. This caused me to have a significant stress reaction which I received treatment for. I felt incredible pressure to provide financially, be a father, support my wife, achieve academically, perform well on clinical placements and keep my business running. It was too much for one person to deal with.

After qualifying as a nurse, I decided to join the RAF as I had always been interested in the military and felt that joining would tick all the boxes. I had aspirations of pre hospital nursing and becoming a MERT (Medical Emergency Response Team) Practitioner. I completed basic training aged 32, the oldest recruit of my intake. This was a test of patience and keeping my head down to get through the nine week course. I was seen as a father figure to many which some aged only 17. I enjoyed this time and also was able to recognise that I was able to spread my wings and not have the burden of a relationship which was problematic and draining. Of course, I missed my son but got to see him at weekends.

I was initially posted to a hospital unit in Lincolnshire where I completed a rotational programme to develop as a newly qualified nurse. This was testing but enjoyable seeing me complete long and tiring shifts which were often emotionally and physically draining. Not long after starting we had our second child after multiple unsuccessful attempts which put added pressure on an already failing marriage. The cracks in the marriage developed subtilty and were hard to see whilst in it. Friends and family could see more clearly but did not push the issue as they wanted the family to work. Hindsight is a wonderful yet useful thing.

PARENTING

Motherhood changed Janet. Almost immediately. I am fully aware that this is quite normal for women, but this change was a complete 180 revealing a completely new personality. She became the subject matter expert on parenting, mostly from Facebook or other unreliable sources, and always knew what the children needed and wanted. I began to be pushed to the wayside and my role was solely the bread winner. Naively, I thought she was acting in the children's best interests and believed what I was told thinking "This must be right as she is their mother and I have to trust her". This became very apparent later down the road not to be the case.

This behaviour started when the children were small. They started sleeping in the marital bed from when they were babies. I was told that this was normal and would help us all have a good night's sleep. This was true in some respect but so unhealthy in others. No child free room, no time to be husband and wife and a relentless flow of children coming through in the night leading to disagreements between us parents about returning them to their own rooms and beds. Speaking with friends I soon found this to be abnormal and, in later years, caused the children significant issues.

My children were now five and three when the third came along. I was happy to have another even if she was not planned. I loved having the children beyond words and did everything I could to provide and be available around work whenever I could. My work saw me complete long and unsociable hours resulting in me getting home exhausted, hungry and in need of some peace and quiet and some food. I was realistic in the understanding that having three young children at home was no walk in the park and wouldn't mind a bit of clutter or mess. Unfortunately Janet felt that the children took complete priority and gave them 100% focus all the time resulting in washing, cleaning, cooking etc to be pushed by the wayside. I would often find myself arriving home to a chaotic, dirty house with dishes stacked up, no food made and the children all up. Even if it was after 8pm. This began to become the common theme. I would often find myself arriving outside the house after work and sitting, waiting, hoping that things would be different tonight and there may be some semblance of order and that I would not enter a house that appeared as if it had been burgled. Unfortunately, this never happened. This was never the fault of the children but of their mother who was unable to stick to routine, get the children to bed on time or, in fact, do or be anywhere on time despite not working.

Bedtimes were, as in most households with young children, interesting. I always thought that the children would become able, as many friends children were, to sleep independently in the knowledge that they were safe and secure in their own beds and rooms. I was again wrong. Janet insisted that we would lie next to each child in turn after a story and wait until they fell asleep. This was the start of an unhealthy, time consuming and difficult routine which ensured the children learned to become more dependent on us, in particular Janet, at bedtime. This combined with getting up in the night and them being allowed to sleep in our bed ensuring no one got a good night's sleep and the children were told that they were allowed to continue to do this by their mother creating increased tension and disagreements between us. I was starting to feel like a visitor in my own home. Something that I never thought would happen. I longed to be part of a team, a united front as a parent and a husband but this never happened despite hoping it would do for years now.

My work saw a move back down south to a nice area by the sea and as my son got older he started in school. Yes! I thought. Finally some structure that the children need which would take the pressure of Janet and free up the time she spent having to look after them. Soon after starting school, Janet reported that he was experiencing difficulties with his peers, concentrating and that he was getting anxious. I felt this to be strange for a boy of such a young age who was bright, happy, active and sociable but I listened and tried to help. These issues were raised with the school by Janet and after a few months I was told that they could not suggest anything else to support him. As I was working full time I had little choice but to run with what Janet had told me and trusted her judgement. She had been researching Home Education and felt that this would suit our son better. She had gone to great lengths researching online the benefits and provided me with lots of articles to read which supported her beliefs.

Janet was incredibly head strong from the beginning and once she had an idea of what she wanted, it would inevitably happen. She was incredibly difficult to reason with and would often fail to grasp very basic concepts and ideas when brought up in discussion leading to unhealthy arguments. I would often, wrongly, simply agree with her for an easy life and to avoid confrontation and which was becoming more frequent. This then spurred her on in other areas of our lives to control and manipulate situations to her liking. Often plans or ideas would change without rationale but simply because she wanted it a certain way. More alarm bells were ringing loud but I put them to the back of my mind, desperate to have a solid family for myself and to provide a stable and loving home for my three awesome children. I did not want them to have to experience a parental separation as I did.

HOME EDUCATING

After much persuasion and being bombarded with one sided articles, I regrettably agreed to trial Home Education for my son. Imagine this. A six year old being home schooled, a three year old causing mayhem and a one year old who was, naturally, needing a lot of looking after. Not a great combination. My son did start in some private classes nearby which were great but failed to provide him with the social, physical and mental challenges that school would offer. They also needed to be paid for which I dutifully obliged despite being on a very modest salary. There were more groups and classes in the surrounding area which kept Janet needed and on hand for him every day with the two younger children in tow. Meanwhile, I was the sole breadwinner and was returning to the house which was becoming more and more disorganised and chaotic as the weeks passed.

Janet loved to be needed and it was quite obvious form an early stage that she prioritised the children above anything else including me and our relationship. She needed to be needed and thrived off appearing to be the best mum out there. Little did she know the very loose foundations she was trying to parent on. She was failing to see the bigger picture of how to raise children and what influence her ideas would have on them later in life. She was making the children become completely dependent on her and causing them to have separation anxiety if they left her side. This was her goal be it conscious or subconscious. She loved that they could not be away from her as it gave her a sense of purpose in her life.

On speaking to friends with children of similar ages, they were continuing to live their lives as parents but also as husbands and wives, going out for dinner and leaving children with relatives regularly for a well needed break and also to keep their marriages healthy and vibrant. This never happened in our situation. No one was allowed to have any say in how the children were raised. Janet took an early dislike to my family, criticising how I was brought up and telling people how strict and unfairly the children were treated when with my family. This was of course untrue. I felt as if I was being isolated from friends and family.

She had had a privileged childhood having been brought up abroad, attending private school and having a housemaid. What became apparent early on in our relationship was how different our views and values were when it came to family. She had a very distant and, soon to be realised, unhealthy relationship with her mother, whom she seemed to actively dislike and avoided spending time with at every opportunity. I, on the other hand, had a close nit family who spoke regularly and had the same healthy values around how to behave and what was acceptable. I felt that Janet was partially jealous of this family network but also had a very liberal approach to parenting so any form of discipline or order was seen in her eyes as wrong. She would often paint me to be authoritarian and strict which was simply untrue. I simply wanted the children to have boundaries and structure to prepare them for life which is essential growing up in the world we live in.

THE BEGINNING OF THE END

This became a reality after an incident whereby I had picked up my middle child, aged 3, carried her upstairs, sat her on her bed and told her off for hitting her little sister. Janet reported this to the local authorities as abuse and that I had in fact thrown my daughter across a room and into a wall. Naturally this ended up with social services making a full investigation with police involvement. This mis management of a normal parenting situation had serious consequences to my career at the time, stopping promotion and preventing me from progressing. This was the start of the end for the marriage as all trust had been broken due to shear lies. I would now start to find out how skewed the system is when it comes to how men are treated. As a man I was immediately guilty and, because of a very believable and manipulative woman, was wrongly labelled. Social services prejudged me by appearance. I am 6ft 3, well built, shaved head and was a keen boxer at the time.

The investigation concluded after a few months and I was found guilty of nothing more than shouting at my child. At this point I should have realised that the marriage was over. There was no trust, plenty of animosity and a continued disagreement of how to parent the three children. The marriage became purely functional. I continued to put my all into it hoping that things would change for the better and we would get back on track. I could not have been more wrong.

A year went by, and my work saw us move again. It was a nice house with a garden, decent neighbours and opposite a primary school. Perfect. We could start the two eldest in a new school fresh. Janet was not in agreement again. She insisted on continuing to educate my son at home and all that that entailed with private lessons and clubs with all the costs associated with them. The middle child started in the primary school but within months there were reports from Janet that there were significant problems. My daughter was refusing to leave the house for school and Janet was unable to get a then five year old into a school which was 200 metres from the front door. Such were the issues that Janet was keen to home educate my daughter in the same way as my son. At the time I was away a lot and could see the issues at home and wrongly agreed for this to happen on a purely trial basis. My daughter was soon taken out of school and started to be home educated. We now had a 8 year old boy and a five year old girl plus a 3 year old all in the house, all day, trying to co-exist. Teaching had to be at three different levels due to age and there were multiple distractions.

I soon found myself dreading coming home after work. It was an unhealthy situation and I highlighted this to Janet on multiple occasions making it clear that my wish was for the children to enter mainstream schooling. The house became even more chaotic and unpleasant to be in. The children were unable to differentiate between being at school and home. It was not working. Despite my wishes, Janet insisted that the children remained home educated. I tried to encourage her to think about the positives of mainstream school but she was adamant that she knew best for the children and dismissed my wishes.

Looking back now It was clear that this was to meet her needs rather than the children. That burning desire to be needed was still strong and Janet was unable to let the children spread their wings without her. This made all three children incredibly clingy and underconfident. They were still unable to sleep independently and it would often be the case that they were all in our bed at night.

At this point in the marriage I was feeling deeply unhappy overwhelmed, claustrophobic, controlled and unable to effect change. In my head the relationship was over. I remember hours on the phone with family and friends over the past few years seeking advice and trying to rationalise my situation. I wanted to leave and had thought about it multiple times over the past five years but was desperate not to upset the children and that I knew that Janet would financially ruin me (which turned out to be true). In my naivety I thought I was protecting them but I was in fact causing them harm by remaining in what had become a toxic relationship with no hope of being fixed.

THE EPIPHANY

In 2019 I found myself working abroad in Africa. My job required me to do this every couple of years. I would miss the children deeply and it would break my heart leaving them each time. I remember driving away from the house with my daughter chasing the car pleading with me not to go. On the other hand I would progressively feel a sense of relief to be away from my marriage. I felt I could truly be myself and not be controlled or manipulated. The real me came out and it was becoming more and more apparent that I had to make a change.

Whilst away I met and worked with an extraordinary women named Alex. There was an instant connection from the off. I remember feeling the electricity between us as soon as we met which was a feeling I had never had before in my life. We instantly hit it off and could spend hours talking about everything and nothing. This was something I had never experienced and this blew my mind to think I had been missing out on being with someone so perfectly matched for me and it had taken a journey of thousands of miles to cross paths. We grew close but unfortunately she nor I were available to each other at the time but from that day forward we spoke daily. Little did I know then but Alex would become a huge part of my life. My time away soon came to an end and I was utterly crushed when I had to say goodbye to her and return to the UK, knowing what lay in store for me. We continued to speak daily when possible and this would be the highlight of my day to hear her voice or see her face on my phone amidst a homelife full of turmoil, conflict and unhappiness.

It was amazing to get back to the children but as soon as I saw Janet, I knew a change was coming. I had no feelings for her anymore. I had had an epiphany whilst I had been abroad after having a lot of time to think about the past and everything that had happened during the marriage. I could not believe what I had put up with. I felt as if I had been controlled and undermined in every aspect of home life. I felt angry with myself beyond belief for putting up with it for so long and wasting the best years of my life.

As a last resort I arranged couples therapy to discuss our issues and try to gain some sort of plan. We were due to move to a new area and I was to start in a new role. The therapy sessions lasted a few weeks but did nothing but highlight the fundamental flaws in our relationship (or what was left of it). The counsellor herself could not believe how we had lasted so long together after hearing our history and at the end of the sessions advised us that one of us would need to make a decision to move forwards as the status quo was not healthy and was damaging the children who were seeing a mother and father who actively disliked one another and who parented in a completely different style with opposite wants and aspirations for the future. Janet openly said that she would not leave me despite this advice and revelation through counselling.

We ended up moving as a family to the new area where I started my new role. The marriage continued to spiral out of control with the house in utter turmoil. There was nothing left. The children were witnessing arguments and were being emotionally harmed by this. It was time to make the hardest yet easiest decision of my life and leave.

I managed to secure a room through work and took with me some basic belongings and set myself up thinking I would come back to collect the rest of my items at a later date. I would soon find out that Janet would never let me back in the family home again nor have access to most of my belongings.

Of course it was upsetting to walk away from your three children, worrying about their reactions and how they would cope. I felt awful in that respect. I felt like I had failed them in every way and was physically sick. On the other hand I had an enormous sensation of a huge weight being taken off my shoulders and I was able to fill my lungs and finally have space to breathe. Such a dichotomy of feelings which were quite overwhelming. I was worried that I would get a sudden urge that I had made the wrong decision but this urge never came. I knew I had a tough journey ahead of me but, again, naively was unaware of how I would be tested….

THE TRANSITION

I dutifully emailed Janet explaining that I was sorry, that we needed for this to happen and that I would happily contribute what was required for the children and for her to enable her to start from fresh. I offered to help with anything she needed and wanted to part on the best of terms to make both our lives and the children's as easy as possible.

I knew there would need to be a fair bit of untangling needed so I contacted a recommended family lawyer for advice. I was sure that the marriage had ended so an application for divorce was made. This was my first encounter with a family solicitor and it was really reassuring to have someone with the correct knowledge and training to help me navigate through, what I thought would be, simple divorce proceedings.

At this time, the Covid 19 pandemic began and the UK saw its first lockdown. This was something new for us all to deal with. Janet immediately restricted my access to the children stating Covid 19 as a reason. I was refused entry back in the house that I was paying for and not allowed to meet with the children face to face. This is where the story really takes a turn….

I was living in a room at work and unable to access my children as I was legally entitled to. Janet would however let me speak to them through a closed window of the family home once a week. She did not let me hug, touch or spend any time alone with them. This was like torture. I was desperate to be able to see them in a natural environment, hug them, take them out for a walk to the park or to play football and to reassure them that I loved them.

I would find myself stood in the rain outside the house I was paying for, full of my own belongings and being refused entry to see my children. What was more worrying was my three children who were normally loving, chatty and tactile with me began to refuse to speak with me through the window. I was broken. I did not know how to fix this situation.

This is where the parental alienation began to raise it's ugly and damaging head.

Cafcass, the government body tasked with assisting the Courts in Children Matter proceedings, defines parental alienation as follows: **"when a child's resistance or hostility towards one parent is not justified and is the result of psychological manipulation by the other parent."**

Soon after in mid-2020, I received letters from Janet's newly appointed solicitor claiming that I should not see the children because of Covid 19. This shortly turned into an accusation that I was not safe to be alone with the children. Janet and I clearly had our polar opposite parenting styles with me being the parent trying to create structure, boundaries and having rules with her having a far more laissez faire approach, letting the children dictate what they did. This obviously created friction within the house. Shortly before leaving the family home, my middle daughter had hurt her younger sister. I had chased after her and shouted at her in response to being worried that she had severely injured her little sister. I placed my hand on my daughters leg whilst telling her off.

I distinctly remember being shopping in Aldi when I received a call from my solicitor who informed me that Janet had again alleged to social services that I was a safeguarding risk to the children and I had chased and hit my daughter leaving a red mark on her leg. I felt the walls come racing inwards and the floor felt like it dropped away. I had to hold onto the shelving to steady myself. I felt sick, my vision blurred, my heart was beating through my neck and I felt as if I was going to be sick. I was utterly shocked. I had not and would never lay a finger on any of my children.

This was the start to the worst two years of my life.

My solicitor now had to deal with the matter of divorce and then needed to commence application for child proceedings to enable me to gain access to my children to whom I was no threat to and had joint responsibility for. I had no other choice than to pay for a professional which was starting to cripple me financially.

Over the years we had jointly bought a property to let out and I had then managed to grow this into four properties. The idea was to give us a steady passive income with a view to finally being able to pay them off and give each child a solid start in life. These jointly owned properties would later be sold and the proceeds used to fund legal fees. The children would now have nothing for their future despite my best intentions and efforts.

Janet had now permitted me, not that she was in a position to give this permission, to see my children face to face in the back garden but to keep two metres distance from them at all times. I had no other way to see them so had to go along with the ludicrous and unlawful request until the case was heard at court. I would arrive at a set time to see the children, in all weather and sit in the garden waiting excitedly to see them. Sometimes they would come outside but often I would be sat on my own with Janet telling me that they did not want to see me and that they were upset as to how I have treated them over the years. This would become her negative narrative of me that she would expose the children to on a daily basis.

One day the children came outside and I walked with them to the park nearby. Janet contacted the police stating I had abducted them. She later refused the children access to my car stating they were unsafe with me.

I felt humiliated, incredibly sad and frustrated being controlled by a scorned individual who had no other motive other than to harm me emotionally and to keep the children dependent of her. Janet was angry, she was clearly upset at being left and this provoked her into acting the way she did. We would later find out that covid was used an a excuse for me not to see my children and that Janet had more deep rooted reasons.

When I left the family home in early 2020 I envisaged difficulties but wanted to have an amicable relationship with Janet for the children's benefit. Her next course of actions would ensure that this would never be possible and that I could and would never be able to forgive her or co-parent.

The children were all at home with Janet and lockdown was in full swing. The youngest had not started school yet and the older two continued to be home educated against my wishes. I had now repeatedly asked, with good reason that they return to mainstream school. Janet point blank refused. The children were now isolated, didn't leave the house and even had home delivery shopping. I was becoming more and concerned for their welfare. It was becoming apparent that Janet and the children were becoming enmeshed and that Janet had actively begun alienating the children from me. This would be proven at a later date.

Multiple court proceedings ensued between May 2020 and ending in November 2022. During this time; a court appointed Clinical Psychologist was directed to make a full assessment of the family. This was partly due to Janet's insistence that the children were unable to enter mainstream school due to them being severely autistic, her accusations of me being mentally unstable and the fact that she was clearly not coping with the situation and alarm bells were ringing with the authorities as to the legitimacy of her claims. It was found that the children were not autistic, that

I was perfectly able to look after and parent my own children and that she in fact had some mental health issues which, combined with malicious intent, were driving her behaviour.

After this; a CAFCASS Guardian was appointed to the children to ensure their best interests were met. They were involved at an early stage, observing my supervised contact with my three children and writing reports and court statements highlighting what would be best for the children.

Supervised contact was initially at my new house and on one occasion, one of Janet's acquaintances acted in that role. This was problematic as they used the opportunity to snoop through my house and belongings, including my bedroom, whilst I spent my very cherished time playing with the kids. This went on for a few months until it was deemed that I did not need to be supervised and I was not a threat to my children. The very fact that this happened due to Janet's false accusations was mortifying. A dad being unable to see his children without supervision, knowing the reasons behind it. Luckily I had very supportive friends and family that made themselves available at short notice, often travelling for hours each weekend to facilitate my contact in adherence with the order.

Contact was then progressed following another hearing and I was able to see the children for a short period of time without supervision. The children began displaying very bizarre and worrying behaviour at handovers. I would often turn up to an agreed location at a court ordered time to collect them or they would be dropped outside my house. Frequently they would refuse to come out of their mothers car, hiding in the boot, covering themselves in coats with little to no encouragement from their mother to attend. I was then asked by Janet to come out to the car to speak to them with her present. This would result in Janet fabricating further abuse allegations on most occasions. I would be accused of speaking, walking, driving, standing, looking in a threatening and aggressive manner. This lead to me deciding against having any contact with her in fear of these allegations sticking. This was someone who was, and is later proven, actively alienating the children from me and exposing them to a constant and harmful negative narrative of me whilst in her care. This ultimately lead to my eldest child vandalising my house, shouting at me, all three children lying and acting in a way in which they had been coached by their mother. They had been told that I was dangerous and that they should be scared of me.

Further observations by social workers and the Guardian happened, all of which were totally positive with the children acting appropriately towards me with hugs, laughter and affection. Finally the professionals were starting to see the reality of this very dangerous situation.

I am in no way guilt free. I had been living in a toxic marriage for many years but felt trapped and unable to leave. I had come from a broken home and desperately wanted my children to not have to experience this. Naively I thought that by staying, I was doing the right thing for them. I was wrong. Towards the end of the marriage, they witnessed multiple arguments and shouting between Janet and me. Janet liked to parent unilaterally and I felt as if I was used for providing a roof over their heads and to fund their lives. Any input I wanted over parenting was shot down and would cause arguments. The children saw this and would side with their mother. I was incredibly frustrated at being undermined and ignored which lead to me shouting at the children and getting cross on a number of times. This was not fair on the children but was a direct result of being trapped in a toxic relationship, being under a huge amount of financial stress as the only earner and feeling undervalued and ignored.

Further court hearings happened and orders were made for contact to happen. Janet continued to break these orders by not turning up at all for handover, arriving late or failing to prepare children or facilitate weekly phone calls with me. The phone calls would either not happen or I would get a child stating they didn't want to talk to me followed by messages from Janet stating that they didn't want to talk due to what I had done to them.

Janet also took it upon herself to engage with the leaders from the children's extra-curricular activities and telling them her version of events. This lead to me almost being assaulted by a group of fathers at an event, witnessed by my child, and some of these individuals believing that the children were at risk from me and that I was not to be near or touch them. This was incredibly distressing and lead to me being unable to attend certain settings in fear of what might happen due to the lies that had been told and believed about me. Janet seemed to have developed a habit of approaching various professionals including charities, GP's and other agencies to tell them her version of events. This would lead to regular safeguarding forms being submitted by these individuals who had unwittingly been manipulated by Janet. It got to the point where the court had to tell Janet to stop doing this as there was no basis of any truth to her allegations and her actions were malicious and unnecessarily reopening issues that had already been dealt with by the judge.

This situation continued with no change. I was living day to day on adrenaline, not sleeping and having work in a particularly demanding and stressful environment. I began to experience episodes of chest pain and started losing clumps of hair due to the amount of stress I was being subjected to. I was also haemorrhaging money on legal fees. I was broke, all my savings had gone trying to see my children. I did the right thing and kept paying Child

Maintenance to Janet for the children leaving me with very little to live off.

The court had ordered the children return to mainstream school in Summer 2021. Janet had protested and disagreed for this to happen citing that she was sufficiently managing their education at home and that the schools were unable to cater for the children's needs. I was relieved, finally places can be secured and the children will be where they can socialise, learn, face adversity, develop, be challenged, enjoy sport, be monitored and gain some independence from their mother. Janet dragged her heels in securing school places and enrolling the children. They finally started in late October unfortunately missing out on the beginning of term in September due to Janet's behaviour. This positive was soon overridden by Janet who was unable to get the children out of the house at all on some days, unable to get them to leave the car at school, would take them out of school unilaterally if she felt there was something more beneficial for them to do and consistently deliver the children with long and dirty hair, often with lice, long dirty finger nails, un ironed clothes and the wrong uniform.

The authorities were becoming more and more concerned as to Janet's ability to parent the children and meet their basic daily needs. My eldest child, who had been out of school the longest, had an incremental reintegration timetable but he would often not go to school and his attendance was below 50%. Janet wanted to slow down his integration and kept brining up autism. This was so frustrating to hear about as I knew there was nothing wrong with the children and the best place for them was school. I was unable to have any effect on this. I would receive regular calls from my eldest child's school asking where he was and that they couldn't get hold of his mother. I would have to explain each time that I could not change the situation whilst they lived with Janet. The Guardian was priceless during this phase and had a direct input in trying to get Janet to ensure the children were in school and holding her accountable for their truancy. This unfortunately did not work. My middle child would hide in the car and refuse to leave at school or refuse to leave the house.

The professionals seemed to be getting to grips with the family dynamic and this was finally highlighted in court. It was found that, yes, I had shouted at my children and that they had witnessed shouting between their parents but that I was not guilty of any physical or mental abuse of them. Nor was I guilty of coercive control, domestic or financial abuse of Janet. It was found that the relationship was a toxic one and that I had done the right thing by moving out of the situation and leaving the marriage to help the children in the future. My time with the children was then increased and I was allowed to have them overnight and without being supported. I was so pleased. I finally felt heard and understood. I thought that this hearing would now pave the way to settled, fair and regular contact.........how I was wrong.

Contact continued to be frustrated by Janet who, amongst other things, would get the children to organise or cancel contact themselves via phone calls or texts, fail consistently to be at point of drop off on time (sometimes just not showing up), would try and have a face to face confrontation in front of the children and requested to meet my new partner (Alex) on her own. One week my eldest did attend contact for a short amount of time having arranged with his mother, without my knowing, that she would pick him up early and would be waiting down the road in her car. This was in clear breach of the court order and was not in their best interest. Before he left, he used the toilet and then left the house. I went to the bathroom to find he had blocked the toilet with loo roll and it was overflowing onto the floor. I went outside to speak to him whilst he was in his mother's car. I was annoyed and appropriately told him off and that his behaviour was not acceptable in my house. His mother soon messaged me stating that my son was scared and that I had acted aggressively and threateningly towards him which was untrue. Each time, Janet would use any situation and make it fit with her negative narrative of me and then document it. I feel that she had told so many lies that she was backed into a corner and had to keep up her story. This happened time and again at handover of the children until I decided I would not approach her car or interact with her in anyway in order to protect myself from her harmful attitude and behaviour.

On another contact session my son had accidentally wet himself whilst playing a game away from the house. He was having fun and didn't want to leave. Janet then documented that he wet himself out of fear and because he had been shouted at.

My daughter had been displaying difficult behaviour and was screaming in the car so much that I decided to pull over. I placed my hand on her leg and told her that she could not continue as it was not safe in the car nor was it reasonable. Janet then created the story that I had hit my daughter causing a red mark on her leg.

Each week I would document failed contact sessions and concerns for the children's welfare and email the Guardian. This happened for over a year. It was so hard seeing my children acting in such an alien way towards me.

STOP THE RIDE, I WANT TO GET OFF

I was exhausted and at my wits end with the whole situation. There was, however, a constant shining light through all of this which kept me sane. Alex. We had kept in daily contact and soon realised that we needed to be together. I had my divorce finalised and she was now in a position to meet. When we did it was just amazing. Everything would stop and I could finally take a breath. She was perfect for me. We connected in every way possible and I knew straight away that I wanted her in my life forever. Luckily she felt the same way.

Towards the end of 2021 I decided to visit her and we spent a couple of weeks together in the sun. It was exactly what we both needed. Towards the end of the trip I proposed to her and thankfully she said yes. It was the easiest question I have ever had to ask. I was ecstatic. This was what all the books and movies where about. We had what everyone is searching for.

I returned to the UK and she soon followed and we began to set up our home together, planning for a wedding in the spring. We were both so happy together. I had no doubts about her. We were such a good team. As a couple, there was nothing we couldn't achieve or cope with. We had many external obstacles to hurdle but both of us felt secure in tackling them due to our rocksteady relationship.

Just as well as a change was afoot.

We married in the spring with friends and family attending from across the world. We both felt so fortunate to be surrounded by so much love and support. It was the complete opposite from my first time round. Chalk and cheese.

BREAKING POINT

Throughout the next few months when contact would happen (or not as was more than not) Janet would message me before, during and after contact. This was incredibly distracting and inappropriate considering I had such limited time with my children. My request for this to stop would fall on deaf ears. These messages became trigger for stress and anxiety.

I continued to lose sleep, have alopecia of my beard and suffered chest pains all of which were investigated and put down to situational stress. As the months went on, I found myself bottling my feelings up as I needed to be strong for the children and continue to attend court without a lawyer due to being broke. The messages and emails continued for a year at which point, after multiple pleas for them to stop, I contacted the police and reported the matter hoping for some assistance. Unfortunately they were unable to action anything as the majority of the messages were linked to the children, even if they were trying to control and manipulate me. I had to block Janet's email and WhatsApp to try and protect myself. I was now down to one sole form of communication with her, an app recommended by social services which could be used for voice calls, messages and video calls. By taking control of the situation and setting boundaries I felt slightly less stressed. I would have physical reactions to messages causing me to shake. The messages were intended to have this effect. The repeated messages and demands to change the contact order (including turning up at children's schools, my house and threatening to turn up at sports clubs) all had the same effect and continue to this day despite multiple requests for them to stop and for us to have no contact unless in case of emergency.

I was Janet's favourite toy and she was not about to let go. The more I ignored her and demonstrated how I had moved on and didn't want her involved in my life, the more she would try and control contact and increase the number of messages she sent.

One of the most worrying parts of this story is that we had shared a large amount of mutual friends prior to separation having been in a long term relationship. Understandingly, it is expected that not all of these friendships would continue but such were the extent and nature of Janet's lies, 99% of these people cut contact and still to this day side with her. This is baffling as Janet had told the world repeatedly for over two years that I had domestically abused her, physically assaulted my children and that I was a real danger to them. I often wonder how these people now compute why, If I was indeed all those things Janet accused me of, the three children were removed from her care and into mine. How had Janet spun her lies to them to fit her narrative? A real mastermind.

I take solace in the fact that I am now free from a controlling and deeply unhappy marriage where I was used as the breadwinner and undermined as a parent. I am now the happiest I have been as an adult, married to Alex who is the love of my life and my best friend, have saved my children from their previous fate, am financially stable and debt free with a career where I have developed experience and specific skills which are highly sought after and are transferable to most industries. My future is bright with unbound potential.

I often look back at my life and curse myself with the "what ifs" and "if only" but I am now a stronger, more resilient person who is able to start their life afresh and live how they want to. I feel that I was meant to go through the last few years hardship and stress to get to where I am now.

THE CHILD MAINTENANCE DISSERVICE

When I left my ex-wife in March 2020 I let her know that I would be happy to pay her directly to help towards the children's daily needs and that I always would. I suggested a figure which seemed reasonable which was immediately dismissed. A few weeks later I received a letter from the CMS who had been contacted by Janet and falsely informed of my income. Janet had purposefully inflated the figure to ensure she received a larger amount. The CMS would not listen to me when I tried to correct this on numerous occasions however when any contact with Janet was had, her word was taken as the truth. Surely, in this day and age, a large agency had moved on from bias towards the female but apparently not. I was met with unhelpful and judgemental case workers who assumed that I was trying to wriggle out of paying for my children. Despite the figure being incorrect, I duly paid what was asked of me immediately to ensure my children were supported. Even then, Janet would ask for more money for the children despite receiving in the region of £900 pcm. I was also paying for the rent and utilities for the children therefore Janet was figuratively living cost free. I attempted to make a change to my CMS payment as I was having to drive initially 2 hrs to see the children but Janet argued and claimed I was lying. Every time I would try and update CMS as to the facts I was dismissed or they would call Janet and she would contradict me and the decision would they be made in her favour.

Fast-forward to July 2022 and the court ordered that the children would move into my full-time care with, initially, very limited daytime contact with their mother. The CMS were updated of the fact but challenged me as I was not receiving the Child Benefit payments (someone else was still claiming for them). They eventually logged that all three children were living with me, full time and without shared care in September 2022. Janet had divulged in court that she was now working and was also claiming benefits. CMS were informed of this multiple times including in written evidence. They made incorrect assessments, changed their minds twice and at the time of writing this they are still under the impression that Janet is not working and that she does not have to pay anything towards the children. I have not received a penny towards the children despite being their main carer and my house being their main residence for the preceding eight months. A formal complaint was made to the CMS who decided to uphold their decision that Janet does not need to contribute anything towards the three children.

All the while this was going on, I was having to incur upwards of £50k of legal fees to try and expose Janet and to get access to see my children and prevent them from being irreparably alienated from me, not having their basic needs catered for, failing to thrive and becoming very mal adjusted humans.

My advice for anyone utilising the CMS is to ensure you send in as much evidence as possible, do not assume they will action anything correctly, be prepared to wait months for anything to be actioned, expect to be on hold for an average of an hour each time you contact them and make sure you hold them to account, double check and complain if necessary. It is not acceptable for an organisation to fail parents this way. I did the right thing by my children but it seems quite easy to be able trick them and then fraudulently not contribute to your own children due to animosity towards the receiving parent.

THE CHANGE

In July 2022 it was ruled that the children would all move into my care full time under a Lives With Order. Janet immediately disputed the decision and appealed to the High Court. This appeal was quickly dismissed and the move went ahead. This was a huge change for us all. The children were all told whilst together by the Guardian at school with me present. It was heart-breaking that we had got to the point that the system had deemed it necessary to move three young children away from their mother and into the care of their father due to non-compliance of multiple child arrangement orders and that their mother was unable to move on with her life and stop denigrating me in front of the children and exposing them to an ongoing negative narrative about me and my life. My youngest had to be physically restrained by me from school and into my car under the supervision of the Guardian. It was the sole worst moment of my life and I was an emotional wreck.

The children were supported appropriately and I did everything I could to help them understand why this was happening to them. Luckily it was summer holidays which gave us a decent amount of time to get used to spending time together and have fun. We also spent time creating a new routine with structure, rules, consequences and boundaries which was a bit of a shock to them considering how they had been living previously. They soon adapted and enjoyed knowing their routine, showering daily, sleeping independently, being lice free, having clean clothes, regular meal and bedtimes. It is crazy but it was a real privilege to have my own children in my house and be able to parent them the way they needed so badly, give them everything they needed and have quality, unmonitored time together. Don't get me wrong there were teething problems with outbursts and some arguing but I remained consistent for them and became their reliable rock.

The summer soon came to an end and it was back to school. This was always a real issue when living with their mother as previously discussed. My eldest had a 49% attendance rate prior to moving to mine. This immediately became 100% come September for all three children. There were no issues getting them into school. They understood very early on that school was not a choice and the importance of being ready on time each day, wearing the right clothes and being clean. Within a matter of days a new routine was established and I could see three happy children attending school, problem free and with good reports from the teachers. What a relief. They were being supported by the schools who had been kept informed throughout proceedings so knew what an ordeal the children had been through. These were three capable children who in no way needed a special education for autism which is what Janet had stated as the main reason to continue to home school against my wishes.

The final court hearing in November 2022 ruled that the three children would remain in my care at my address and have a schedule of limited contact with their mother for the proceeding ten months with every other weekend overnight stays. Finally my name had been cleared and I was deemed to be the parent most capable of meeting all three children's needs and ensuring contact with the other parent would take place as ordered. It was a huge relief. My life needed to change in many aspects to allow me to be the parent the children needed. I had managed to secure a larger house and, after much time and effort, got my employer to agree flexible working to allow me to drop off and pick up form school. I had finally done it, the children would now be given the opportunity to live a normal live and thrive.

I thought that I would now be able to relax and focus on living my new life with my wife and children but my brain had other ideas. I started having more anxiety leading to shaking episodes which would last for days at a time. My sleep deteriorated to the point where I needed to be prescribed benzodiazepines to get some rest in order to function the next day. I began to feel at capacity all of the time and that I was just about staying afloat. I got support through the Dr and was referred for talking therapy. This initially helped but my symptoms returned and got progressively worse. I was experiencing Post Traumatic Stress according to the professionals. Trauma of being in a controlling marriage for a decade followed by three years of intense stress where I had almost lost my children, job, house, income and when I had to act as my own barrister on multiple occasions against top London barristers being paid thousands. These events had taken their toll on my health and I needed time off to rebuild.

My work were very supportive and allowed me time off sick whilst I received therapy and started new medications to help me sleep and boost my mood and capacity for life. I was then able to spend time healing, time outside with the dog, surfing, exercising, reading and writing this book.

I took charge of my mental health after recognising that I was not well. Understanding that you are having difficulties and asking for help is the first but most important step. Had I not engaged with my doctor or utilised debt charities (after being signposted by a friend who had been in a similar situation) then I would be in a completely different situation. I was also incredibly fortunate to have a very supportive family and social circle who kept me accountable and helped me to remain objective throughout the last few years.

If you are finding yourself reading this and seeing similarities with your own situation then I urge you to reach out for some help. It is impossible to navigate life's problems alone even when mentally strong.

Things always appear worse at night, when you reassess in the daytime your worries lessen. This is where the journalling comes in useful. Keep a book by your bed to write down all you thoughts when you can't sleep. This helped me no end.

What have I learnt from the last few years? Be honest. The truth will always prevail and justice will be served. Be true to yourself. Work hard at becoming the best version of you that you can. Be kind to yourself no matter what. You have the power to change your life for the better one small step at a time.

I hope that this story has highlighted how no matter how bad the situation is, things will improve.

You will be ok in the end.

STEPS I TOOK TO IMPROVE MY MENTAL HEALTH

1. Cold showers - Every morning lasting 90 seconds – proven to boost mood and increase metabolism.

2. Exercise – A change in the type of training I did encompassing whole body workouts using weights, boxing and running – this had a much greater effect than working out one body part at a time.

3. Dog walking – twice daily walks with the dog. A walk first thing in the morning would clear my head and ensure I was fresh for the day. The dog was a purchase by my wife who promptly left the country for work for two months! I was left with three children and a puppy. The puppy is now a dog and the best companion you could ask for. Animals are incredibly healing. Combine this with talking to friends whilst walking and you have a recipe for positivity.

4. Journalling – Keeping a journal each day and keeping it by my bed so when I woke up in the night I was able to write down what was on my mind, helping me get back to sleep.

5. Headspace App – This was invaluable on long nights when I couldn't sleep. I would do a meditation before bed and listen to sleep stories in the night.

6. Surfing – I had surfed a little when I was younger but decided that this activity would be something I could start to focus on. It enable me to switch off from the world, use my body and mind together and also be exposed to the elements. The cold shock during January is really mind blowing. I still walk away from a session like I have been reborn. Nothing beats the high of catching a wave and

nothing cleanses your brain like the shock of being in a freezing cold washing machine when you wipe out.

7. Talking – My friends and family have been pivotal in keeping me sane throughout the last few years, in particular my elder brother whom I am forever indebted to. Talking helps you sound out your issues and get another perspective which often ends up making the situation seem less dark.

USEFUL POINTS OF CONTACT

www.stepchange.org

Their team of debt experts help hundreds of thousands of people a year to deal with their debt problems.

www.nhs.uk

The first place to look for simple health advice and for signposting to where you can access help.

www.citizensadvice.org.uk

Online free advice from Citizens Advice to help you find a way forward, whatever the problem.

www.headspace.com

Everyday Mindfulness and Meditation for Stress, Anxiety, Sleep, Focus, Fitness, and More.

www.mind.org.uk

Support minds – offering help whenever you might need it through their information, advice and local services.

www.samaritans.org

Get in Touch About Anything That's Troubling You No Matter How Big or Small the Issue Is. They're Here to Help You Work Through What's on Your Mind.